D1785669

Step-By-Step
Instant Pot Cookbook

Instant Pot Recipes with Step-by-Step
Procedures, Best Meals Ever For Living a Life full
of Energy and Lose your Weight in Health!

Brian Smith

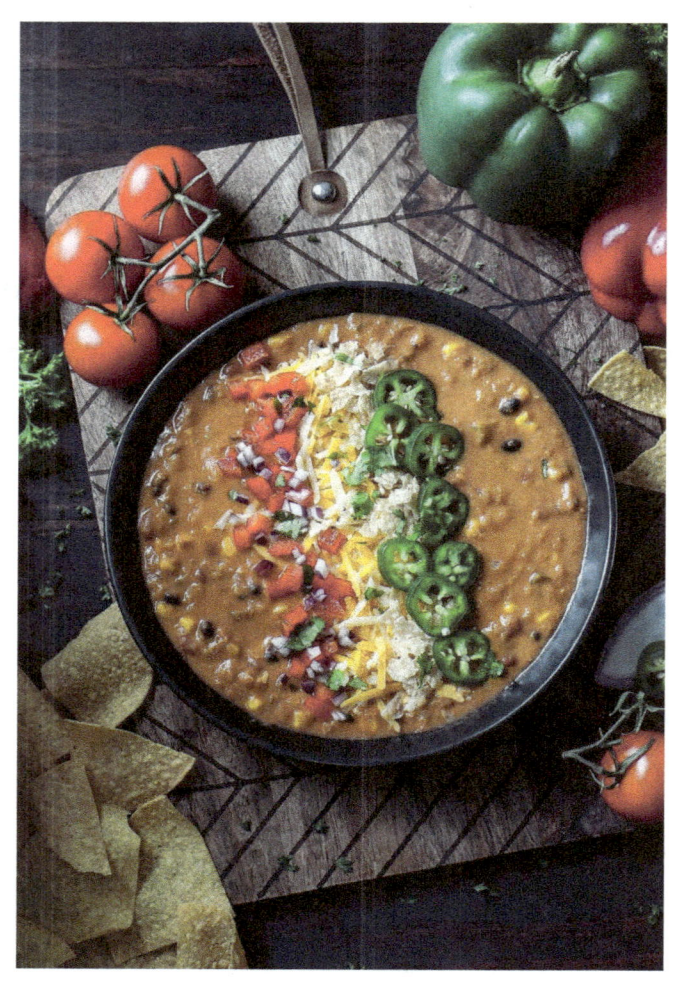

Table of Contents

© Copyright 2021 by Brian Smith - All rights reserved. The following Book is reproduced below with the goal of providing information that is as accurate and reliable as possible. Regardless, purchasing this Book can be seen as consent to the fact that both the publisher and the author of this book are in no way experts on the topics discussed within and that any recommendations or suggestions that are made herein are for entertainment purposes only. Professionals should be consulted as needed prior to undertaking any of the action endorsed herein. This declaration is deemed fair and valid by both the American Bar Association and the Committee of Publishers Association and is legally binding throughout the United States. Furthermore, the transmission, duplication, or reproduction of any of the following work including specific information will be considered an illegal act irrespective of if it is done electronically or in print. This extends to creating a secondary or tertiary copy of the work or a recorded copy and is only allowed with the express written consent from the Publisher. All additional right reserved. The information in the following pages is broadly considered a truthful and accurate account of facts and as such, any inattention, use, or misuse of the information in question by the reader will render any resulting actions solely under their purview. There are no scenarios in which the publisher or the original author of this work can be in any fashion deemed liable for any hardship or damages that may befall them after undertaking information described herein. Additionally, the information in the following pages is intended only for informational purposes and should thus be thought of as universal. As befitting its nature, it is presented without assurance regarding its prolonged validity or interim quality. Trademarks that are mentioned are done without written consent and can in no way be considered an endorsement from the trademark holder.

Introduction

Instant pot is a pressure cooker, also stir-fry, stew, and cook rice, cook vegetables and chicken. It's an all-in-one device, so you can season chicken and cook it in the same pan, for example. In most cases, instant pot meals can be served in less than an hour.

Cooking less time is due to the pressure cooking function that captures the steam generated by the liquid cooking environment (including liquids released from meat and vegetables), boosts the pressure and pushes the steam back.

But don't confuse with traditional pressure cookers. The instant pot, unlike the pressure cooker used by grandparents, eliminates the risk of safety with a lid that locks and remains locked until pressure is released.

Even when cooking time is over in the instant pot, you need to take an additional step-to release the pressure.

There are two ways to relieve pressure. Due to the natural pressure release, the lid valve remains in the sealing position and the pressure will naturally dissipate over time. This process takes 20 minutes to over an hour, depending on what is cooked. Low fluidity foods (such as chicken wings) take less time than high fluidity foods such as soups and marinades.

Another option is manual pressure release (also called quick release). Now you need to carefully move the valve to the ventilation position and see that the steam rises slowly and the pressure is released. This Directions is much faster, but foods with high liquid content, such as soups, take about 15 minutes to manually relieve pressure.

Which option should I use? Take into account that even if natural pressure is released, the instant pot is still under pressure. This means that the food will continue to cook while the instant pot is in sealed mode. Manual pressure relief is useful when the dishes are well cooked and need to be stopped as soon as possible.

If the goal is to prepare meals quickly, set the cooking time for dishes that are being cooked in an instant pop and release the pressure manually after the time has passed.

Instant pots (called "Instapot" by many) are one of our favorite cookware because they can handle such a wide range of foods almost easily. Instant pots range from those that work on the basics of pressure cooking to those that can be sterilized using Suicide video or some models can be controlled via Wi-Fi.

In addition, if you want to expand the range of kitchenware, the Instant Pot brand has released an air fryer that can be used to make rotisserie chicken and homemade beef jerky. There is also an independent accumulator device that can be used in instant pots to make fish, steaks and more.

The current icon instant pot works like a pressure cooker and uses heat and steam to quickly cook food. Everything from perfect carnitas to boiled eggs was cooked, but not all ingredients and DIRECTIONSs work. Here are few foods that should not be cooked in classic instant pots.

Instant pots are not pressure fryer and are not designed to handle the high temperatures required to heat cooking oils like crispy fried chicken. Of course, the instant pot is great for dishes like Carnitas, but after removing the meat from the instant pot, to get the final crispness in the meat, transfer it to a frying pan for a few minutes or to an oven top and hot Crispy in the oven.

As with slow cookers, dairy products such as cheese, milk, and sour cream will pack into instant pots using pressure cooking settings or slow cooking settings. Do not add these ingredients after the dish are cooked or create a recipe in Instapot.

There are two exceptions. One is when making yogurt. This is merely possible if you are using an instant pot recipe. The other is only when making cheesecake and following an instant pot recipe.

Although you can technically cook pasta in an instant pot, gummy may appear and cooking may be uneven. To be honest, unless you have a choice, cooking pasta in a stove pot is just as fast and easy and consistently gives you better cooked pasta.

Instead of baking the cake in an instant pot, steam it. The cake is moist-it works for things like bread pudding-but there is no good skin on the cake or on the crunchy edge everyone fights with a baked brownie. However, let's say your desire is to build a close-up or a simple dessert with your family; you can get a damp sponge in about 30 minutes, except during the DIRECTIONS time.

Canning, a technique for cooking and sealing food in a jar, is often done in a pressure cooker. Therefore, it is recommended to create a batch of jam, pickles or jelly in Instapot. Please do not.

With an instant pot, you can't monitor the temperature of what you can, like a normal pressure cooker. In canning, it is important to cook and seal the dishes correctly. Incorrect cooking and sealing can lead to the growth of bacteria that can cause food poisoning.

If you want to avoid canning in an instant pot, some newer models, such as Duo Plus, have a sterilization setting that can clean kitchen items such as baby bottles, bottles and cookware.

Instant Pot Pressure Cooker Safety Tips

Instant Pot is a very safe pressure cooker consisting of various safety mechanisms. do not worry. It will not explode immediately. Most accidents are caused by user errors and can be easily avoided. To further minimize the possibility of an accident, we have compiled a list of safety tips.

1 Don't leave it alone

It is not recommended to leave home while cooking an instant pot. If you have to leave it alone, make sure it is under pressure and no steam is coming out.

2 Do not use KFC in instant pot

Do not fry in an instant pot or other pressure cooker.

KFC uses a commercial pressure fryer specially made to fry chicken (the latest one that operates at 5 PSI). Instant pots (10.5-11.6 PSI) are specially made to make our lives easier.

3 water intake!

Instant pots require a minimum of 1 1/2 cup liquid (Instant Pot Official Number) 1 cup liquid to reach and maintain pressure.

The liquid can be a combination of gravy, vinegar, water, chicken etc.

4 half full or half empty

The max line printed on the inner pot of the instant pot is not for pressure cooking.

For pressure cooking: up to 2/3 full

Food for pressure cooking that expands during cooking (grains, beans, dried vegetables, etc.): up to 1/2

5 Not a facial steamer

Deep cleaning is not performed even if the pressure cooker steam is used once.

When opening, always tilt the lid away from you. Wear waterproof and heat-resistant silicone gloves especially when performing quick release.

6 never use power

In situations of zero, you should try to force open the lid of the instant pot pressure cooker, unless you want to prevent a light saber from hitting your face.

7 Wash Up & Checkout

If you want to be secured, wash the lid after each use and clean the anti-block shield and inner pot. Make sure that the gasket (silicon seal ring) is in good shape and that there is no food residue in the anti-block shield before use.

Usually silicone seal rings should be replaced every 18-24 months. It is always advisable to keep extra things.

Do not purchase a sealing ring from a third party because it is an integral part of the safety features of the instant ring. Using sealing rings that have not been tested with instant pot products can create serious safety concerns."

Before use, make sure that the sealing ring is securely fixed to the sealing ring rack and the anti-block shield is properly attached to the vapor discharge pipe.

A properly fitted sealing ring can be moved clockwise or counterclockwise in the sealing ring rack with little force.

With instant pots, the whole family can cook meals in less than 30 minutes. Cooked dishes such as rice, chicken, beef stew, sauce, yakitori can be cooked for 30-60 minutes from the beginning to the end. And yes, you can bake bread in an instant pot.

Old and ketogenic diet fans love instant pots for their ability to `` roast " meat in such a short time, but vegetarians and vegans that can quickly cook dishes such as pumpkin soup, baked potatoes and marinated potato chilis, also highly appreciated oatmeal cream and macaroni and cheese.

Even dried beans, which usually require overnight cooking, can be prepared in 30 minutes to make spicy hummus.

Beef with Pineapples, Raisins, and Pistachios

Preparation Time: 20 minutes

Cooking Time: 75 minutes

Servings: 2

Ingredients:

30 oz. beef, ground

1 cup of pistachios

1 cup of pineapples, diced

1 cup of dried raisins, chopped

2 medium onions, peeled and chopped

6 cloves garlic, minced

2 teaspoons chili powder

3 teaspoons oregano

1 teaspoon cumin powder

5 tablespoons olive oil

2 cups of tomatoes, chopped

2 cups of chicken broth

2 teaspoons nutmeg

Salt and pepper to taste

Directions:

Rinse and soak the raisins in the warm water for 10 minutes and then set aside.

Combine the oregano, nutmeg, cumin, pistachios, garlic, salt, and black pepper. Season the beef with the spice mix. Then set the beef aside to marinate for at least a few hours unrefrigerated at room temperature or in the fridge overnight.

Put the instant potto SAUTE mode and add the olive oil to heat it.

Fry the chopped onions for around 10 minutes until caramelized.

Add the ground beef and stir for 5 minutes, breaking the beef.

SAUTE until fragrant, then spoon all the remaining ingredients and mix well.

Make sure to lock the lid and cook for50 minutes on a HIGH PRESSURE and then release the pressure over 10 minutes.

Serve with the white wine and enjoy!

Nutrition:

Calories – 376

Fat – 75 g

Carbs – 26.1 g

Protein – 57 g

Instant Goose with Herbs and Madeira

Preparation Time: 10 minutes

Cooking Time: 45 minutes

Servings: 2

Ingredients:

1 goose, cut into pieces

1 cup of Madeira wine (or other fortified wine)

2 carrots, peeled and diced

2 potatoes, peeled and diced

2 tablespoons soy sauce

1 tablespoon dry basil

2 tablespoons cilantro

2 tablespoons rosemary

2 tablespoons oregano

2 tablespoons thyme

5 garlic cloves, minced

4 tablespoons olive oil

2-3 teaspoons salt

1 cup of water

Directions:

Toss the goose pieces into the salt, soy sauce, dry basil, minced garlic, cilantro, rosemary, oregano, and thyme. Pour the Madeira in and marinate the goose for at least 10 hours unrefrigerated at room temperature or place in the fridge overnight.

Add the marinated goose and all the listed ingredients to your Instant Pot. Make sure to lock the lid and fix the timer to 45 minutes and cook the duck on MEAT/STEW mode.

Naturally release the pressure over 10 minutes.

Portion the goose into two plates and dollop each plate with the cooking liquid and soya sauce. This dish should be served warm. Serve the goose with the buckwheat on the side if you prefer.

Nutrition:

Calories – 357

Fat – 64 g

Carbs – 26.7 g

Protein – 59 g

Flavorful Spaghetti

Preparation Time: 5 minutes

Cooking Time: 20 minutes

Servings: 4

Ingredients:

6 oz spaghetti noodles

2 tbsp parmesan cheese

1 1/4 cups chicken stock

2 tbsp tomato paste

1 cup jar spaghetti sauce

1/2 tsp dried oregano

1/2 tsp dried basil

1 garlic clove, minced

1/2 onion, diced

1/2 lb ground beef

1 tbsp olive oil

1/2 tsp salt

Directions:

Set instant pot on sauté mode and olive oil into the pot.

Add ground beef and sauté for 3 minutes, stir and break meat with a spoon.

Add onion and cook for 4 minutes.

Stir in garlic, oregano, basil, spaghetti sauce, chicken stock, tomato paste, parmesan cheese, pepper, and salt. Stir well.

Turn off the pot. Break noodles in half and add layer them in the meat mixture.

Seal instant pot with lid and select pressure cook mode and set the timer for 8 minutes.

Once the timer goes off then release pressure using quick release method than open the lid.

Stir well to combine.

Serve and enjoy.

Nutrition:

Calories 594

Fat 18.4 g

Carbohydrates 57.9 g

Sugar 6 g

Protein 48.1 g

Cholesterol 167 mg

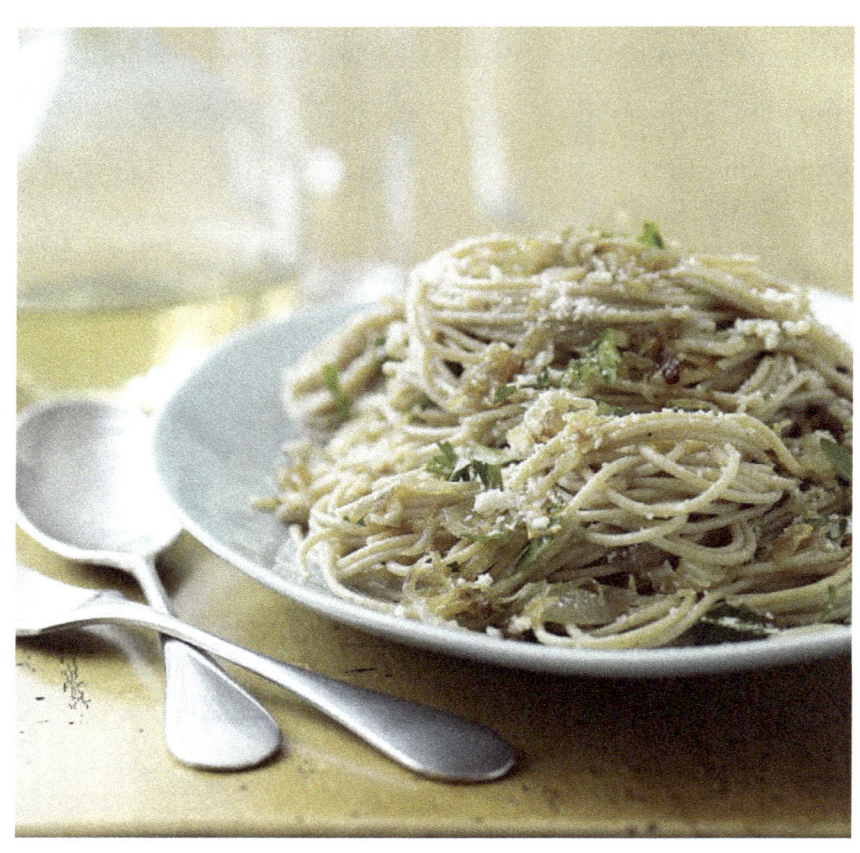

Jerk Chicken & Rice

Preparation Time: 5 minutes

Cooking Time: 15 minutes

Servings: 4

Ingredients:

2 chicken thighs, skinless and boneless

1 cup chicken broth

1 tbsp jerk seasoning

1 garlic clove, minced

1/2 small onion, diced

3/4 cup long grain rice, rinsed

2 tsp olive oil

Directions:

Set instant pot on sauté mode. When instant pot display reads hot then add olive oil.

Add onion and sauté for few minutes or until onion softens.

Add garlic and sauté for 20 seconds. Stir constantly.

Add jerk seasoning and stir well to mix.

Add rice and chicken broth and stir well. Now add the chicken.

Seal instant pot with lid and select pressure cook mode and set the timer for 7 minutes.

Allow to release pressure naturally for 5 minutes then release using quick release method than open the lid. Stir well and serve.

Nutrition:

Calories 599

Fat 16.7 g

Carbohydrates 58.1 g

Sugar 1.2 g

Protein 49.9 g

Cholesterol 130 mg

Tasty Cream Cheese Risotto

Preparation Time: 5 minutes

Cooking Time: 15 minutes

Servings: 4

Ingredients:

2 1/2 cups Arborio rice

6 oz cream cheese, softened

1/2 cup pecans, chopped

1 tbsp pepper

2 tbsp fresh lemon juice

1 cup white wine

5 cups chicken broth

2 tbsp garlic, minced

2 onions, chopped

4 tbsp olive oil

Directions:

Add olive oil into the instant pot and set the pot on sauté mode.

When the display reads hot then add onions and garlic and sauté for 3 minutes.

Stir in wine and rice and cook until wine absorbed.

Add broth and stir well. Seal pot with lid and select high pressure for 6 minutes.

Allow to release pressure naturally then open the lid.
Season with pepper and lemon juice and stir in cream cheese.

Garnish with chopped pecans and serve.

Nutrition:

Calories 566

Fat 18.1 g

Carbohydrates 78.4 g

Sugar 4.6 g

Protein 15.1 g

Cholesterol 5 mg

Easy Coconut Rice

Preparation Time: 5 minutes

Cooking Time: 15 minutes

Servings: 4

Ingredients:

2 cups rice, soaked and drained

1/2 cup fresh coriander leaves, chopped

1 cup unsweetened coconut, grated

1 tbsp cinnamon powder

1/4 tbsp cloves

1/2 cup currants

4 tbsp olive oil

4 cups vegetable stock

1 tbsp salt

Directions:

Add olive oil into the instant pot and set the pot on sauté mode.

Add cloves and cinnamon powder into the pot and sauté for 30 seconds.

Add rice and stir well. Add remaining ingredients and cook for 1 minute.

Seal pot with lid and cook on high for 6 minutes.

Allow to release pressure naturally then open the lid.

Stir well and serve.

Nutrition:

Calories 538

Fat 21.4 g

Carbohydrates 79.2 g

Sugar 2.4 g

Protein 7.5 g

Cholesterol 0 mg

Chicken Cheese Pasta

Preparation Time: 5 minutes

Cooking Time: 15 minutes

Servings: 4

Ingredients:

1 lb chicken breasts, skinless, boneless, and cut into chunks

2 tbsp parmesan cheese

1 1/2 cups cheddar cheese, shredded

1/2 tbsp mustard

1 cup hot water

3/4 cup heavy cream

8 oz pasta

2 tbsp butter

1/2 tbsp olive oil

1/4 tsp pepper

1/2 tsp sea salt

Directions:

Add olive oil into the instant pot and set the pot on sauté mode.

When instant pot display reads hot then add chicken chunks and sauté for 4-5 minutes.

Add remaining ingredients except for cheeses and heavy cream. Stir well.

Seal pot with lid and select high pressure for 12 minutes.

Allow to release pressure naturally then open the lid.

Now set the pot on sauté mode and add cheddar cheese, parmesan cheese, and heavy cream. Stir well until cheese is melted.

Serve and enjoy.

Nutrition:

Calories 650

Fat 35.6 g

Carbohydrates 33.3 g

Sugar 0.1 g

Protein 47.1 g

Cholesterol 220 mg

Tasty Cheeseburger Macaroni

Preparation Time: 5 minutes

Cooking Time: 15 minutes

Servings: 3

Ingredients:

1/2 lb ground beef

1 cup elbow macaroni, uncooked

1/2 tsp basil

1/2 onion, chopped

1 1/2 cups chicken broth

1/2 cup cheddar cheese, shredded

1 tbsp Italian seasoning

14 oz can tomatoes, diced

7.5 oz can tomato sauce

1 1/2 tsp garlic, minced

1/2 tbsp seasoning salt

Directions:

Set instant pot on sauté mode.

When instant pot display reads hot then add onion and ground beef and sauté until meat is no longer pink.

Add garlic, seasoning salt, Italian seasoning, and basil and sauté for 5 minutes.

Add tomatoes, tomato sauce, and broth and stir well.

Add macaroni in and stir well. Seal pot with lid and select high pressure for 4 minutes.

Release pressure using quick release method than open the lid.

Stir in cheese and serve.

Nutrition:

Calories 408

Fat 13.6 g

Carbohydrates 34.9 g

Sugar 9.9 g

Protein 36.1 g

Cholesterol 91 mg

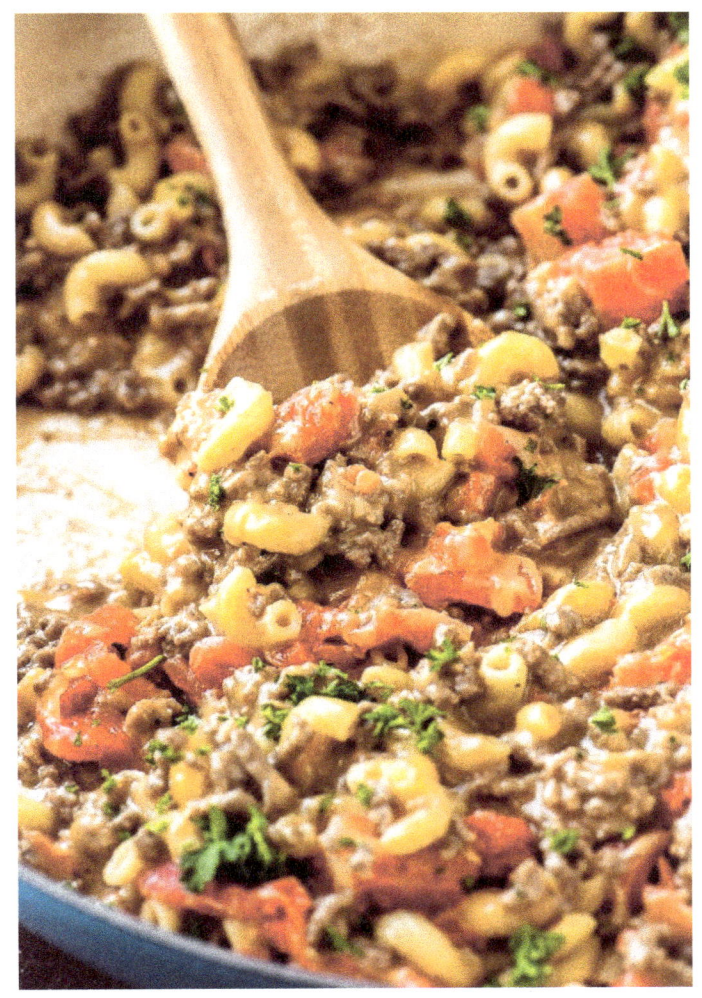

Quick Cheese Macaroni

Preparation Time: 5 minutes

Cooking Time: 10 minutes

Servings: 3

Ingredients:

1/2 lb pasta

6 oz evaporated milk

1/2 cup mozzarella cheese, grated

1/2 cup cheddar cheese, shredded

16 oz chicken broth

Pepper

Salt

Directions:

Add broth and pasta into the instant pot. Seal pot with lid and select high pressure for 5 minutes.

Release pressure using quick release method than open the lid.

Add milk and cheese and stir until pasta is coated. Season with pepper and salt.

Serve and enjoy.

Nutrition:

Calories 407

Fat 14 g

Carbohydrates 48.1 g

Sugar 6.2 g

Protein 21.5 g

Cholesterol 94 mg

Delicious Creamy Ziti

Preparation Time: 5 minutes

Cooking Time: 15 minutes

Servings: 4

Ingredients:

1/2 cup mozzarella cheese, shredded

1 cup parmesan cheese, shredded

1 cup pasta sauce

8 oz ziti pasta

1 tsp garlic, minced

1 cup heavy cream

1 1/2 cups chicken broth

Pepper

Salt

Directions:

Add chicken broth, heavy cream, garlic, pepper, salt, and noodles to the instant pot.

Seal pot with lid and select high pressure for 6 minutes.

Allow to release pressure naturally then open the lid.

Add pasta sauce and stir well. Slowly add cheese and stir until cheese melt and sauce thicken.

Serve and enjoy.

Nutrition:

Calories 430

Fat 20.7 g

Carbohydrates 41.9 g

Sugar 5.8 g

Protein 18.6 g

Cholesterol 100 mg

Perfect Alfredo

Preparation Time: 5 minutes

Cooking Time: 15 minutes

Servings: 4

Ingredients:

1/2 lb dry linguine noodles, break in half

3/4 cup parmesan cheese, shredded

1 tsp garlic, minced

1 1/2 cups heavy cream

1 1/2 cups vegetable broth

Pepper

Salt

Directions:

Add vegetable broth, heavy cream, garlic, pepper, salt, and noodles to the instant pot.

Seal pot with lid and select high pressure for 6 minutes.

Release pressure using quick release method than open the lid.

Add parmesan cheese and stir until cheese melted.

Serve and enjoy.

Nutrition:

Calories 279

Fat 22.8 g

Carbohydrates 7.7 g

Sugar 0.6 g

Protein 11.2 g

Cholesterol 76 mg

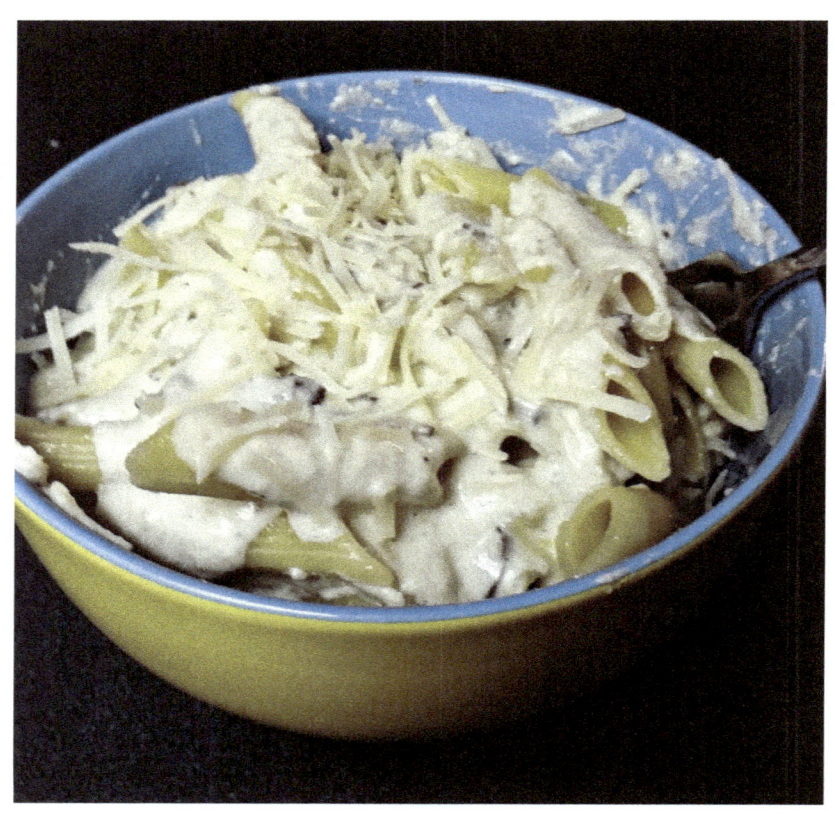

Simple Tomato Rice

Preparation Time: 5 minutes

Cooking Time: 15 minutes

Servings: 4

Ingredients:

1 cup rice, soaked and drained

3 tbsp olive oil

1 cup water

1 tbsp cumin seeds

8 tomatoes, sliced

1/2 tsp pepper

1/2 tbsp salt

Directions:

Add olive oil into the instant pot and set the pot on sauté mode.

When instant pot display reads hot then add cumin seeds and sauté for 30 seconds.

Add tomatoes and sauté for 6 minutes. Add rice, pepper, and salt and stir well.

Seal pot with lid and select high pressure for 6 minutes.

Allow to release pressure naturally then open the lid.

Stir well and serve.

Nutrition:

Calories 413

Fat 15.5 g

Carbohydrates 63.2 g

Sugar 8.8 g

Protein 7.7 g

Cholesterol 0 mg

Mushroom Pea Risotto

Preparation Time: 5 minutes

Cooking Time: 25 minutes

Servings: 4

Ingredients:

1/2 cup Arborio rice

2 tbsp parmesan cheese, grated

1/4 cup frozen peas, thawed

1 cup baby spinach

1/8 tsp dried thyme

1 cup chicken broth

4 oz cremini mushrooms, sliced

1/2 onion, diced

1 garlic clove, minced

2 tbsp butter

Pepper

Salt

Directions:

Add 1 tablespoon of butter into the instant pot and set the pot on sauté mode.

Once butter is melted then add onion and garlic and sauté for 2-3 minutes.

Add mushrooms and cook until tender, about 3-4 minutes. Season with pepper and salt.

Add broth, thyme, and rice and stir well. Seal pot with lid and select high pressure for 6 minutes.

Release pressure using quick release method than open the lid.

Add spinach and remaining butter and stir until spinach is wilted about 2 minutes.

Stir in parmesan cheese and peas, about 1 minute.

Serve hot and enjoy.

Nutrition:

Calories 239

Fat 9.3 g

Carbohydrates 31.4 g

Sugar 2.3 g

Protein 7.3 g

Cholesterol 23 mg

Vegetable Parmesan Risotto

Preparation Time: 5 minutes

Cooking Time: 20 minutes

Servings: 4

Ingredients:

1 1/2 cups Arborio rice

1 tbsp butter

1/2 lemon juice

1 tbsp parsley, chopped

1/2 onion, chopped

3 garlic cloves, minced

1/2 cup dry white wine

3 1/2 cups chicken broth

5 asparagus, sliced

1 cup fresh spinach

2 tsp olive oil

1/2 cup parmesan cheese, shredded

1 lb shrimp, peeled and deveined

Pepper

Salt

Directions:

Add 1 tsp olive oil into the instant pot and set the pot on sauté mode.

Add asparagus and cook for 2-3 minutes or until softened. Remove asparagus from pot and set aside. Add garlic and onion and sauté for a minute.

Add butter and melt. Add rice and stir for 1-2 minutes. Add white wine and stir well.

Add broth and parmesan. Stir. Season with pepper and salt.

Seal pot with lid and select high pressure for 8 minutes. Release pressure using quick release method than open the lid.

Set instant pot on sauté mode. Move risotto to one side of the pot.

Now add remaining oil to other side then add veggies and shrimp. Cook shrimp for 3-4 minutes or until shrimp are pink.

Add spinach and cook until wilted. Stir everything well in the pot.

Drizzle with lemon juice and sprinkle with chopped parsley.

Serve and enjoy.

Nutrition:

Calories 551, Fat 11.5 g, Carbohydrates 63.3 g

Sugar 1.8 g, Protein 39.5 g Cholesterol 254 mg

Parmesan Shrimp Risotto

Preparation Time: 5 minutes

Cooking Time: 25 minutes

Servings: 4

Ingredients:

1 lb shrimp, peeled, deveined, and chopped

1/2 cup parmesan cheese, grated

1 cup clam juice

3 cups chicken broth

1/4 cup dry sherry

1 1/2 cups Arborio rice

1 tbsp paprika

1 tbsp oregano leaves, minced

1 roasted red pepper, chopped

1 onion, chopped

2 tbsp butter

1/2 tsp black pepper

1/2 tsp salt

Directions:

Add butter into the instant pot and set pot on sauté mode.
Once butter is melted then add onion and roasted pepper
and cook for 4 minutes.

Stir in the oregano, pepper, paprika, and salt and cook for a minute.

Add rice and stir for a minute. Add sherry and cook until absorbed.

Add clam juice and broth. Stir. Seal pot with lid and select high pressure for 10 minutes.

Release pressure using quick release method than open the lid.

Set pot on sauté mode and add shrimp and stir until shrimp is cooked about 2 minutes.

Serve and enjoy.

Nutrition:

Calories 600

Fat 14.1 g

Carbohydrates 71.2 g

Sugar 4.7 g

Protein 41.5 g

Cholesterol 269 mg

Basil Tomato Risotto

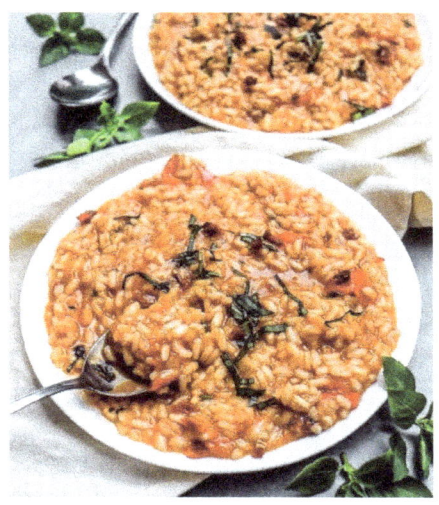

Preparation Time: 5 minutes

Cooking Time: 15 minutes

Servings: 4

Ingredients:

1 1/2 cups Arborio rice

1 tbsp dried basil

1 cup cherry tomatoes, cut in half

3 tbsp basil pesto

2 cups vegetable stock

1 onion, diced

1 tbsp butter

1 tbsp olive oil

1/2 tsp salt

Directions:

Add butter and oil into the instant pot and set the pot on sauté mode.

Add onion and sauté until softened. Add Arborio rice and cook for 3-5 minutes.

Add stock, pesto, and salt. Stir well.

Seal pot with lid and select high pressure for 5 minutes.

Release pressure using quick release method than open the lid.

Add tomatoes, parmesan, and basil and stir until well combined.

Serve and enjoy.

Nutrition:

Calories 356

Fat 9.6 g

Carbohydrates 62.7 g

Protein 5.7 g

Cholesterol 8 mg

Healthy Veggie Pasta

Preparation Time: 5 minutes

Cooking Time: 15 minutes

Servings: 3

Ingredients:

1 cup vegetable stock

1/2 bell pepper, chopped

1 cup spinach, chopped

1/2 tomato, diced

1/2 medium yellow squash, chopped

1/2 small onion, diced

12 oz pasta sauce

6 oz spiral pasta

Directions:

Add vegetables, pasta sauce, and stock and stir well.

Seal pot with lid and select high pressure for 4 minutes.

Allow to release pressure naturally then open the lid.

Stir well and serve.

Nutrition:

Calories 325

Fat 4.9 g

Carbohydrates 62.2 g, Sugar 13.1 g

Protein 11.2 g, Cholesterol 2 mg

Poultry

Kung Pao Chicken

Preparation Time: 5 minutes

Cooking Time: 17 minutes

Servings: 5

Ingredients:

Coconut oil – 2 tbsps.

Boneless, skinless chicken breasts – 1 pound, cubed

Hot sauce – 6 tbsps.

Cashews – ½ cup, chopped

Ginger – ½ tsp. finely grated

Chili powder – ½ tsp.

Kosher salt – ½ tsp.

Freshly ground black pepper – ½ tsp.

Directions:

Press Sauté add oil and heat it. Add chicken, salt, pepper, chili powder, ginger, cashews, and hot sauce. Make sure to lock the lid and Press Manual. Cook on High for 17 minutes.

Nutrition:

Calories – 380,Protein – 30.6 g. ,Fat – 25 g. ,Carbs – 7 g.

Whole Roast Chicken

Preparation Time: 10 minutes

Cooking Time: 25 minutes

Servings: 6

Ingredients:

Butter – 4 tbsps.

Dried basil – 1 tsp.

Dried cilantro – 1 tsp.

Salt – ½ tsp.

Black pepper – ½ tsp.

Bone broth – ½ cup

Whole chicken – 1

Directions:

In a bowl, mix the butter, salt, pepper, basil, and cilantro. Add bone broth into the IP. Brush the chicken with the butter mixture and place into the IP (keep the breast facing the bottom of the pot). Cover and cook 25 minutes on Meat settings. Do a natural pressure release. Remove chicken, carve and enjoy.

Nutrition:

Calories – 215

Protein – 21.6 g.

Fat – 13.4 g., Carbs – 1 g.

Chicken Cacciatore

Preparation Time: 5 minutes

Cooking Time: 18 minutes

Servings: 4

Ingredients:

Coconut oil – 6 tbsps.

Chicken legs – 5

Bell pepper – 1, diced

Dried basil – ½ tsp.

Onion – ½, chopped

Dried parsley – ½ tsp.

Salt – ½ tsp.

Freshly ground black pepper – ½ tsp.

Diced tomatoes – 1 (14-ounce) can

Directions:

Press Sauté and melt the oil. Add the chicken and sauté until browned. Remove chicken and set aside. Add tomatoes, black pepper, salt, parsley, onion, basil, and pepper and sauté. Add ½-cup water and add the chicken on top. Make sure to lock the lid and hit Cancel. Press Manual and cook on High for 18 minutes. Do a natural release and serve. **Nutrition:** Calories – 344,Protein – 26.5 g. ,Fat – 24.3 g. ,Carbs – 5 g.

Spicy Mexican Chicken

Preparation Time: 5 minutes

Cooking Time: 17 minutes

Servings: 4

Ingredients:

Avocado oil – 2 tbsps.

Chicken – 1 pound, ground

Finely chopped jalapeno – ½

Coriander – ½ tsp.

Crushed red pepper – ½ tsp.

Curry powder – ½ tsp.

Chili powder – ½ tsp.

Salt – ½ tsp.

Freshly ground black pepper – ½ tsp.

Poblano chili pepper – ¼ finely chopped

Tomatoes – 1 (14 ounces) can

Directions: Press Sauté and heat the oil. Add ½-cup water, then add tomatoes, chili pepper, black pepper, salt, chili powder, curry powder, red pepper, coriander, jalapeno, and chicken. Make sure to lock the lid and hit Cancel. Press Manual and cook 17 minutes on High. Do a natural release. Open and serve. **Nutrition:** Calories – 269,Protein – 30 g. ,Fat – 14.7 g. ,Carbs – 4.2 g.

Turkey Burger with Fries

Preparation Time: 5 minutes

Cooking Time: 10 minutes

Servings: 4

Ingredients:

Coconut oil 2 tbsps.

Bacon – 6 slices

Thinly sliced avocado – 1

Turkey – ½ pound, ground

Freshly ground black pepper – ½ tsp.

Parsley – ½ tsp. dried

Turmeric – ½ tsp. ground

Dried basil – ½ tsp.

Salt – ½ tsp.

Broccoli – 2 cups, chopped

Water – ¼ cup

Directions:

Spread an aluminum foil. On top of the foil wrap the bacon around the avocado slices. Fold the foil to make a packet. In a bowl, mix turkey, salt, basil, turmeric, parsley, and black pepper. Combine and make a large and thin patty. Press Sauté and add oil in your IP. Add ¼-cup water into the Instant Pot. Place in the patty and broccoli. Insert the trivet and place the aluminum foil packet on top. Close and press Manual. Cook for 10 minutes on High. Do a natural release. Open and remove the food. Cut the patty in 4 parts. Serve with avocado fries.

Nutrition:

Calories – 429

Protein – 29.4 g.

Fat – 31.5 g.

Carbs – 8.1 g.

Spicy Turkey Meatballs

Preparation Time: 10 minutes

Cooking Time: 25 minutes

Servings: 5

Ingredients:

Ground turkey – 1 pound

Hot sauce – ¼ cup

Coconut oil – 2 tbsps.

Grated ginger – 1 tsp.

Chili powder – ½ tsp.

Basil – ½ tsp. dried

Salt – ½ tsp.

Ground black pepper – ½ tsp.

Directions:

Make 1 ½ inch meatballs with the ground turkey and place in a dish. In a bowl, stir together salt, pepper, basil, chili powder, ginger, oil, and hot sauce. Mix and sprinkle evenly over the meatballs. Add 1 cup water into the Instant Pot and insert the trivet. Gently place the meatball dish on top of the trivet. Close and press Manual. Cook 25 minutes on high. Do a natural pressure release. Open and serve. **Nutrition:** Calories – 205,Protein – 26.7 g. ,Fat – 10.1 g. ,Carbs – 0.7 g.

Cheesy Chicken with Jalapenos

Preparation Time: 5 minutes

Cooking Time: 12 minutes

Servings: 4

Ingredients:

Chicken breasts – 1 pound

Cheddar cheese – 8 ounces, grated

Sour cream – ¾ cup

Jalapenos – 3, seeded and sliced

Water – ½ cup

Cream cheese – 8 ounces

Salt and pepper to taste

Directions:

In the IP, whisk together the water, sour cream, and cheeses. Mix in the jalapenos and place the chicken inside. Flavor with salt and pepper. Make sure to lock the lid and cook on Manual for 12 minutes. Do a quick release. Serve.

Nutrition:

Calories – 310

Protein – 20 g.

Fat – 26 g.

Carbs – 4 g.

Creamy Bacon Chicken

Preparation Time: 10 minutes

Cooking Time: 30 minutes

Servings: 4

Ingredients:

Cream cheese – 8 ounces

Bacon slices – 8, cooked and crumbled

Chicken breasts – 2 pounds

Ranch seasoning – 1 packet

Cheddar cheese – 4 ounces, shredded

Arrowroot – 2 tbsps.

Water – 1 cup

Directions:

Whisk together the water, cream cheese and seasoning in the Instant Pot. Add the chicken breast. Make sure to lock the lid and cook on High for 25 minutes. Choose Cancel and use a quick pressure release. Put the chicken to a cutting board and shred with forks. Press sauté and stir in the arrowroot. Add bacon, shredded chicken, and cheddar. Cook for about 3 to 4 minutes, or until thickened. Serve.

Nutrition:

Calories – 620Protein – 48 g. ,Fat – 38 g. ,Carbs – 6 g.

Italian Duck with Spinach

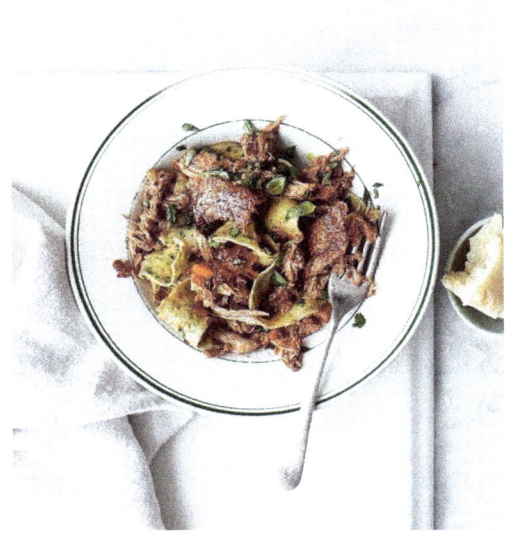

Preparation Time: 5 minutes

Cooking Time: 15 minutes

Servings: 3

Ingredients:

Duck breasts – 1 pound, halved

Spinach – ½ cup, chopped

Chopped Sun-Dried Tomatoes – ¼ cup

Chicken stock – ½ cup

Grated Parmesan Cheese – ¼ cup

Italian seasoning – 1 tsp.

Heavy cream – 1/3 cup

Minced garlic – 1 tsp.

Salt and pepper to taste

Olive oil – 2 tbsps.

Directions:

Whisk together the seasoning, garlic, oil, and salt and pepper. Brush this mixture to the meat. Lay the duck in the IP and cook on Sauté until golden completely. Add the stock, Make sure to lock the lid and cook on Manual for 4 minutes. Press Cancel and do a quick release. Stir in the remaining ingredients and cover. Cook on High for 5 minutes more. Release the pressure quickly and serve.

Nutrition:

Calories – 455

Protein – 57 g.

Fat – 26 g.

Carbs – 1 g.

Creamy Mushroom Turkey

Preparation Time: 10 minutes

Cooking Time: 30 minutes

Servings: 10

Ingredients:

Turkey breast – 1 ¼ pounds

White wine – 1/3 cup

White button mushrooms – 6 ounces, sliced

Arrowroot – 1 tbsp.

Garlic – 1 clove, minced

Minced shallots – 3 tbsps.

Olive oil – 2 tbsps.

Parsley – ½ tsp.

Chicken stock – 2/3 cup

Heavy cream – 3 tbsps.

Directions: Tie the turkey every 2 inches, crosswise. Press Sauté and heat the oil in it. Add the turkey and brown on all sides. Set aside. Add the garlic, mushrooms, shallots, and parsley. Cook for a few minutes. Add the broth and return the turkey to the pot. Cook on High for 15 minutes. Do a quick pressure release. Transfer the turkey to a plate. Untie and slice it. Whisk the cream and arrowroot in the Instant Pot and cook until thickened. Drizzle the sauce over the turkey. Serve.

Nutrition:

Calories – 192

Protein – 25 g.

Fat – 15 g.

Carbs – 4.5 g.

Soft and Juicy Chicken

Preparation Time: 10 minutes

Cooking Time: 30 minutes

Servings: 10

Ingredients:

Chicken – 1 (4-pound)

Coconut oil – 1 tbsp.

Lemon juice – 2 tbsps.

Garlic – 2 cloves, peeled

Paprika – 1 tsp.

Chicken stock – 1 ½ cups

Salt – ½ tsp.

Pepper – ¼ tsp.

Onion powder – 1 tsp.

Directions:

In a bowl, combine all the spices. Rub the mixture into the chicken. Add the coconut oil in the IP and melt on Sauté. Add the chicken and cook until browned on all sides. Pour the lemon juice and stock over. Add the garlic cloves. Close and cook on Manual for 25 minutes. Serve.

Nutrition:

Calories – 270

Protein – 22 g. ,Fat – 20 g. ,Carbs – 3 g.

Herby Juicy Chicken Fillets

Preparation Time: 5 minutes

Cooking Time: 13 minutes

Servings: 4

Ingredients:

Olive oil – 2 tbsps.

Chicken fillets – 4

Red wine – ¼ cup

Chicken broth – ¾ cup

Ground black pepper and salt to taste

Dried marjoram – ½ tsp.

Dried sage – 1 tsp.

Dried parsley flakes – ½ tsp.

Dried basil – ½ tsp.

Directions:

Press Sauté and add oil to the Instant Pot. Sear chicken for about 8 minutes. Turning once or twice. Add the red wine and deglaze the pot. Add the rest of the ingredients. Cover and cook on Poultry for 5 minutes on High. Do a natural release and serve.

Nutrition:

Calories – 357,Protein – 43.2 g. Fat – 18.4 g. ,Carbs – 1 g.

Chicken Bowl with Pine Nuts

Preparation Time: 5 minutes

Cooking Time: 20 minutes

Servings: 4

Ingredients:

Chicken legs – 1 pound, skinless and cut into pieces

Olive oil – 1 tbsp.

Red wine vinegar – 2 tbsps.

Watercress – 1-ounce, tough stalks removed and chopped

Bell pepper – 1, chopped

Sweet onion – 1, sliced

Garlic – 2 cloves, minced

Cucumber – 1, sliced

Gem lettuce – 2 cups, leaves separated

Ground black pepper and salt to taste

Spanish paprika – 1 tsp.

Marjoram – ½ tsp.

Oregano – ½ tsp.

Pine nuts – 4 tbsps.

Water – 1 cup, for the pot

Directions:

Add 1 cup water and a metal rack to the Instant Pot. Lower the chicken legs onto the metal rack. Cover and cook on Steam mode for 15 minutes on High. Do a quick release and open. Slice the chicken into bite-sized pieces and discard the bones. Place the meat into a bowl. Clean the Instant Pot and add 1 tbsp. oil. Heat on Sauté. Add sweet onion and garlic and sauté for 5 minutes. Put in the rest of the ingredients except for the pine nuts and lettuce and mix. Add the mixture to the bowl and toss to combine. Garnish with pine nuts and serve with lettuce leaves.

Nutrition:

Calories – 328

Protein – 24.7 g.

Fat – 20.6 g.

Carbs – 11.1 g.

Chicken with Asparagus & Jasmine Rice

Preparation Time: 10 minutes

Cooking Time: 40 minutes

Servings: 4

Ingredients:

1 tbsp olive oil

4 chicken breasts

1 tsp garlic salt

½ cup onion, finely diced

2 garlic cloves, minced

1 cup jasmine rice

1 lemon, zested and juiced

2 ¼ cups chicken broth

1 cup asparagus, chopped

1 tbsp parsley for garnish

Black pepper to taste

Lemon slices to garnish

Directions:

Set to Sauté, heat olive oil, season chicken with garlic salt and black pepper, and sear until golden brown, 6 minutes; set aside. Put the onion in and cook until softened, 3 minutes. Stir in garlic, allow to release fragrant for 30 seconds.

Stir in rice and cook until translucent, 3 minutes. Add lemon zest, lemon juice, broth, asparagus, salt, pepper, and place chicken on top. Seal the lid, Choose Pressure Cook on High, and set time to 5 minutes. After cooking, perform natural release for 15 minutes. Unlock the lid, fluff rice, and plate. Garnish with parsley and lemon slices to serve.

Nutrition:

Calories – 646

Protein – 88 g.

Fat – 25 g.

Carbs – 22 g.

Chicken with Rotini, Mushrooms & Spinach

Preparation Time: 10 minutes

Cooking Time: 30 minutes

Servings: 4

Ingredients:

2 tbsp butter

4 chicken breasts, cut into cubes

Salt and black pepper to taste

1 small yellow onion, diced

2 cups sliced white mushrooms

1 garlic clove, minced

1 lb rotini pasta

6 cups chicken broth

1 tsp chopped oregano

4 cups chopped baby spinach

½ cup crumbled goat cheese

Directions:

Set to Sauté, melt butter, season chicken with salt and pepper, and sear until golden brown, 4 minutes; set aside in a plate. Put the onion and mushrooms in and cook until softened, 4 minutes. Stir in garlic, for 30 seconds. Return chicken to pot, stir in rotini, broth, and oregano. Seal the lid, Choose Pressure Cook on High, and set time to 3 minutes.

Once done cooking, do a natural pressure release for 10 minutes. Choose Sauté and unlock the lid. Stir in spinach, allow wilting, and mix in goat cheese until adequately incorporated. Adjust taste with salt, black pepper, and serve warm.

Nutrition:

Calories – 687

Protein – 63 g.

Fat – 32 g.

Carbs – 35 g.

Thai Chicken Curry Rice

Preparation Time: 10 minutes

Cooking Time: 35 minutes

Servings: 4

Ingredients:

4 chicken thighs

Salt and black pepper to taste

2 tbsp olive oil

2 medium carrots, julienned

1 red bell pepper, thinly sliced

2 tbsp red curry paste

1 garlic clove, minced

1 tsp ginger paste

1 cup basmati rice

1 ½ cups chicken broth

1 cup coconut milk

1 lime, cut into wedges to garnish

Directions:

Set to Sauté, heat olive oil, season chicken with salt and pepper, and sear until golden brown on both sides, 6 minutes; set aside. Add carrots and bell pepper to oil and cook until softened, 4 minutes. Stir in curry paste, garlic, and ginger; sauté for 1 minute. Add rice, broth, coconut milk and give ingredients a good stir. Arrange chicken on top. Seal the lid, select Manual/Pressure Cook on High, and set time to 10 minutes. After cooking, do a natural release for 10 minutes. Unlock the lid, fluff rice, and adjust the taste. Garnish with lime wedges and serve.

Nutrition:

Calories – 715

Protein – 43 g.

Fat – 48 g.

Carbs – 38 g.

Rich Louisiana Chicken with Quinoa

Preparation Time: 5 minutes

Cooking Time: 20 minutes

Servings: 4

Ingredients:

2 tbsp olive oil

4 chicken breasts, thinly sliced

1 tsp Creole seasoning

2 green bell peppers, sliced

1 cup dry rainbow quinoa

2 cups chicken broth

Salt to taste

1 lemon, zested and juiced

2 chives, chopped

Directions:

Set to Sauté, heat olive oil, season chicken with Creole seasoning, and fry with bell peppers until chicken is golden brown on both sides, 5 minutes and peppers soften. Stir in quinoa, broth, and salt. Seal the lid, Choose Pressure Cook on High, and set time to 1 minute. After cooking, do a quick pressure release, and press Sauté. Fluff quinoa, and stir in lemon zest, lemon juice, and chives. Dish meal into bowls and serve warm with hard-boiled eggs.

Nutrition:

Calories – 523

Protein – 37 g.

Fat – 17 g.

Carbs – 32 g.

Spicy Chicken Manchurian

Preparation Time: 10 minutes

Cooking Time: 35 minutes

Servings: 4

Ingredients:

½ cup olive oil

4 tbsp cornstarch, divided

2 eggs, beaten

2 tbsp soy sauce, divided

Salt and black pepper to taste

4 chicken breasts, cubed

2 tbsp sesame oil

1 tbsp fresh garlic paste

1 tbsp fresh ginger paste

1 red chili, sliced

2 tbsp hot sauce

½ tsp honey

1 cup chicken broth

2 scallions, sliced for garnishing

Directions:

Set to Sauté and heat olive oil. Whisk cornstarch, eggs, soy sauce, salt, and pepper. Pour chicken into mixture and stir to coat well. Fry coated chicken until golden brown on all sides, 8 minutes. Put it on top of a paper towel-lined plate to drain grease. Empty inner pot, wipe clean with a paper towel and return to base.

Heat in sesame oil and sauté garlic, ginger, and red chili until fragrant and chili softened, 1 minute. Stir in hot sauce, honey, broth, and arrange chicken in sauce. Seal the lid, Choose Pressure Cook mode on High, and set time to 3 minutes. After cooking, do natural pressure release for 10 minutes. Spoon into bowls and garnish with scallions.

Nutrition:

Calories – 722

Protein – 61 g.

Fat – 46 g.

Carbs – 14 g.

Honey-Lemon Chicken with Vegetables

Preparation Time: 10 minutes

Cooking Time: 40 minutes

Servings: 4

Ingredients:

4 skin-on, bone-in chicken legs

2 tbsp olive oil

Salt and black pepper to taste

4 cloves garlic, minced

1 tsp fresh chopped thyme

½ cup dry white wine

1 ¼ cups chicken stock

1 cup carrots, chopped

1 cup parsnip, chopped

3 tomatoes, chopped

1 tbsp honey

4 slices lemon

Fresh thyme, chopped for garnish

Directions:

Season the chicken with pepper and salt. Warm oil on Sauté mode. Arrange chicken legs into the hot oil; cook for 3 to 5 minutes each side until browned. Place in a bowl and set aside.

Sauté thyme and garlic in the chicken fat for 1 minute until soft and lightly golden.

Add wine into the pot to deglaze, scrape the pot's bottom to get rid of any brown bits of food. Simmer the wine for 2 to 3 minutes until slightly reduced in volume. Add stock, carrots, parsnip, tomatoes, pepper and salt into the pot. Lay steam rack onto veggies.

Into the pressure cooker's steamer basket, arrange chicken legs. Set the steamer basket onto the rack. Drizzle the chicken with honey then top with lemon slices.

Make sure to lock the lid and cook on High Pressure for 12 minutes. Release Pressure naturally for 10 minutes.

Place the chicken to a bowl. Drain the veggies and place them around the chicken. Garnish with fresh thyme before serving.

Nutrition:

Calories – 700

Protein – 58 g.

Fat – 40 g.

Carbs – 17 g.

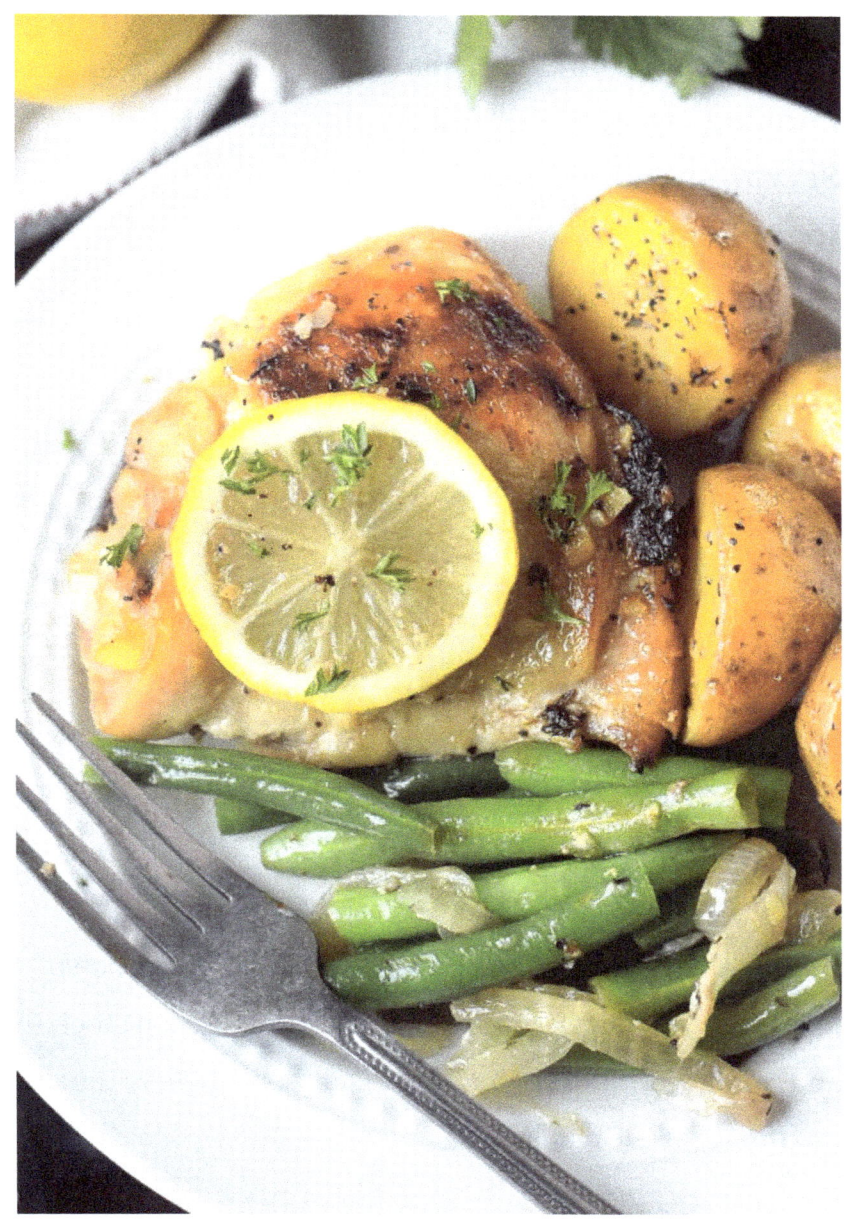

Sweet & Citrusy Chicken Breasts

Preparation Time: 10 minutes

Cooking Time: 30 minutes

Servings: 4

Ingredients:

2 chicken breasts, cubed

½ cup honey

½ cup orange juice

1/3 cup soy sauce

1/3 cup chicken stock

1/3 cup hoisin sauce

1 garlic clove, minced

2 tsp cornstarch

2 tsp water

1 cup diced orange

3 cups hot cooked quinoa

Directions:

Organize the chicken at the bottom of the pot. In a bowl, mix honey, soy sauce, garlic, hoisin sauce, chicken stock, and orange juice, until the honey is dissolved. Pour the mixture over the chicken.

Make sure to lock the lid and cook on High Pressure for 7 minutes. Release the pressure quickly. Take the chicken from the pot and set to a bowl. Press Sauté. In a small bowl, mix water with cornstarch. Pour into the liquid within the pot and cook for 3 minutes until thick. Stir diced orange and chicken into the sauce until well coated. Serve with quinoa.

Nutrition:

Calories – 680

Protein – 53 g.

Fat – 36 g.

Carbs – 16 g.

Savory Orange Chicken

Preparation Time: 15 minutes

Cooking Time: 50 minutes

Servings: 6

Ingredients:

2 tbsp olive oil

6 chicken breasts, boneless, skinless, cubed

1/3 cup chicken stock

¼ cup soy sauce

2 tbsp brown sugar

1 tbsp lemon juice

1 tbsp garlic powder

1 tsp chili sauce

1 cup orange juice

Salt and black pepper to taste

2 cups cooked gnocchi

Directions:

Warm oil on Sauté. In batches, sear chicken in the oil for 5 minutes until browned. Set aside in a bowl.

In your pot, mix orange juice, chicken stock, sugar, chili sauce, garlic powder, lemon juice, and soy sauce; Stir in chicken to coat. Make sure to lock the lid and cook on High Pressure for 7 minutes. Release the Pressure quickly.

Take ¼ cup liquid from the pot to a bowl; stir in cornstarch to dissolve; mix into sauce in the pot until the color is consistent. Press Sauté and cook sauce for 5 minutes until thickened. Season with pepper and salt. Serve the chicken with gnocchi.

Nutrition:

Calories – 710

Protein – 62 g.

Fat – 42 g.

Carbs – 24 g.

White Wine Chicken Breasts with Fresh Herbs

Preparation Time: 5 minutes

Cooking Time: 15 minutes

Servings: 4

Ingredients:

4 boneless, skinless chicken breasts

½ tsp salt

1 cup water

¼ cup dry white wine

½ tsp rosemary, chopped

½ tsp mint, chopped

½ tsp marjoram, chopped

½ tsp sage, chopped

Directions

Dash salt over the chicken and put it in the pot. Mix in mint, rosemary, marjoram, and sage. Pour wine and water around the chicken. Close the pot, and cook for 6 minutes on High Pressure. Naturally release the pressure for 10 minutes.

Nutrition:

Calories – 650,Protein – 49 g. ,Fat – 31 g. ,Carbs – 10 g.

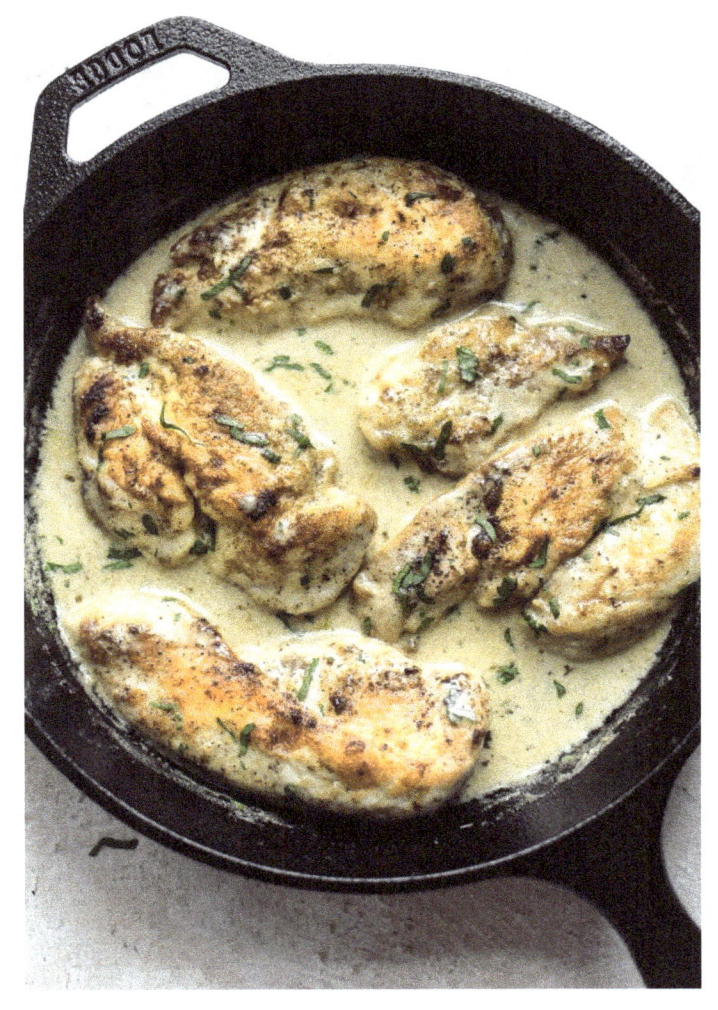

Crispy Bacon & Bean Chicken

Preparation Time: 15 minutes

Cooking Time: 45 minutes

Servings: 4

Ingredients:

1 tbsp olive oil

4 slices bacon, crumbled

4 boneless, skinless chicken thighs

1 onion, diced

4 garlic cloves, minced

1 tbsp tomato paste

1 tbsp oregano

1 tbsp ground cumin

1 tsp chili powder

½ tsp cayenne pepper

1 (14.5-ounce) can whole tomatoes

1 cup chicken broth

1 tsp salt

1 cup cooked corn

1 red bell pepper, chopped

1 cup shredded Monterey Jack cheese

1 cup chopped red onion

15 oz red kidney beans, rinsed

¼ cup chopped cilantro

Directions:

Warm oil on Sauté. Sear the chicken for 3 minutes for each side until browned. Set the chicken on a plate. In the same oil, fry bacon until crispy, about 5 minutes and set aside.

Add in onion, red onion, and cook for 3 minutes until fragrant. Stir in garlic, oregano, cayenne, cumin, tomato paste, bell pepper, and chili, and cook for 30 more seconds. Pour the chicken broth, salt, and tomatoes and bring to a boil. Take back the chicken and bacon to the pot and ensure it is submerged in the braising liquid.

Make sure to lock the lid and cook on High Pressure for 15 minutes. Release the Pressure quickly. Pour the corn and kidney beans in the cooker, Press Sauté and bring the liquid to a boil; cook for 10 minutes. Serve topped with shredded cheese and chopped cilantro.

Nutrition:

Calories – 750

Protein – 71 g.

Fat – 55 g.

Carbs – 33 g.

Delicious Pulled Chicken with Peach Sauce

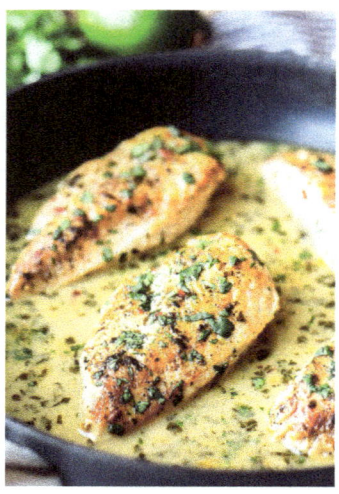

Preparation Time: 10 minutes

Cooking Time: 40 minutes

Servings: 4

Ingredients:

15 ounces canned peach chunks

4 boneless, skinless chicken thighs

14 ounces canned diced tomatoes

2 cloves garlic, minced

½ tsp cumin

½ tsp salt

Cheddar shredded cheese

Fresh chopped mint leaves

Directions:

Strain canned peach chunks. Reserve the juice and set aside. In your instant pot, add chicken, tomatoes, cumin, garlic, peach juice (about 1 cup), and salt. Seal the lid, press Poultry and cook on High for 15 minutes. Do a quick Pressure release. Shred chicken with the use of two forks. Transfer to a serving plate. Add peach chunks to the cooking juices and mix until well combined. Pour the peach salsa over the chicken, top with chopped mint leaves and shredded cheese. Serve immediately.

Nutrition:

Calories – 720

Protein – 64 g.

Fat – 47 g.

Carbs – 22 g.

Chicken & Quinoa Soup

Preparation Time: 10 minutes

Cooking Time: 30 minutes

Servings: 6

Ingredients:

2 tbsp butter

1 cup red onion, chopped

1 cup carrots, chopped

1 cup celery, chopped

2 boneless, skinless chicken breasts, cubed

4 cups chicken broth

6 ounces quinoa, rinsed

1 tbsp fresh parsley, chopped

Salt and black pepper to taste

4 oz mascarpone cheese, at room temperature

1 cup milk

1 cup heavy cream

Directions:

Melt butter on Sauté. Add onion, celery, and carrots then cook for 5 minutes until tender.

Add broth, mix in parsley, quinoa and chicken. Season with pepper and salt.

Make sure to lock the lid and cook on High Pressure for 5 minutes. Release the pressure quickly. Press Sauté.

Add mascarpone cheese to the soup and stir well to melt completely; mix in heavy cream and milk. Let the soup simmer for 3 to 4 minutes until thickened and creamy.

Nutrition:

Calories – 530

Protein – 37 g.

Fat – 26 g.

Carbs – 8 g.

Okra & Rice Chicken with Spring Onions

Preparation Time: 10 minutes

Cooking Time: 25 minutes

Servings: 4

Ingredients:

6 garlic cloves, grated

¼ cup tomato puree

½ cup soy sauce

1/3 cup honey

2 tbsp rice vinegar

1 tbsp olive oil

4 boneless, skinless chicken breasts, chopped

1 cup rice, rinsed

½ tsp salt

2 cups water

2 cups frozen okra

1 tbsp cornstarch

1 tbsp water

2 tsp toasted sesame seeds

4 spring onions, chopped

Directions:

In the pot, mix garlic, tomato puree, vinegar, soy sauce, honey, and oil; toss in chicken to coat. In an ovenproof bowl that can fit in the instant pot, mix water, salt and rice.

Set the steamer rack on top of chicken. Lower the bowl onto the rack. Make sure to lock the lid and cook on High Pressure for 10 minutes. Release the pressure quickly. Use a fork to fluff the rice. Lay okra onto the rice. Allow the okra steam in the residual heat for 3 minutes.

Take the trivet and bowl from the pot. Set the chicken to a plate. Press Sauté. In a small bowl, mix a tablespoon of water and cornstarch until smooth. Stir into the sauce and cook for 3 to 4 minutes until thickened. Divide the rice, chicken, and okra between 4 bowls. Drizzle sauce over each portion; garnish with spring onions and sesame seeds.

Nutrition:

Calories – 730

Protein – 65 g.

Fat – 47 g.

Carbs – 32 g.

Macaroni with Chicken & Pesto Sauce

Preparation Time: 10 minutes

Cooking Time: 30 minutes

Servings: 8

Ingredients:

3 ½ cups water

4 chicken breast, boneless, skinless, cubed

8 oz macaroni pasta

1 tbsp butter

Salt and black pepper to taste

2 cups fresh collard greens, trimmed

1 cup cherry tomatoes, halved

½ cup basil pesto sauce

¼ cup cream cheese, at room temperature

1 garlic clove, minced

¼ cup asiago cheese, grated

Freshly chopped basil for garnish

Directions:

Add water, chicken, 2 tsp salt, butter, and macaroni, and stir well to mix and be submerged in water. Make sure to lock the lid and cook for2 minutes on High Pressure. Release the Pressure quickly. Press Cancel, open the lid, get rid of ¼ cup water from the pot.

Set on Sauté mode. Into the pot, mix in collard greens, pesto sauce, garlic, remaining 1 teaspoon salt, cream cheese, cherry tomatoes, and black pepper. Cook for 1 to 2 minutes as you stir, until sauce is creamy. Place the pasta into serving plates. Top with asiago cheese and basil before serving.

Nutrition:

Calories – 760

Protein – 74 g.

Fat – 51 g.

Carbs – 41 g.

Mouthwatering Green Salsa on Chicken Breasts

Preparation Time: 10 minutes

Cooking Time: 40 minutes

Servings: 4

Ingredients:

Salsa Verde:

1 jalapeño pepper, deveined and chopped

½ cup capers

¼ cup parsley

1 lime, juiced

1 tsp salt

¼ cup extra virgin olive oil

Chicken:

4 boneless skinless chicken breasts

2 cups water

1 cup quinoa, rinsed

Directions:

In a blender, mix olive oil, salt, lime juice, jalapeño pepper, capers, and parsley and blend until smooth. Organize chicken breasts at the bottom of the cooker. Over the chicken, add salsa verde mixture.

In a bowl that can fit in the cooker, mix quinoa and water. Set a steamer rack onto chicken and sauce. Set the bowl onto the rack. Make sure to lock the lid and cook on High Pressure for 20 minutes. Release the Pressure quickly. Remove the quinoa bowl and rack. Using two forks, shred chicken into the sauce; stir to coat. Divide the quinoa, between plates. Top with chicken and salsa verde before serving.

Nutrition:

Calories – 690

Protein – 56 g.

Fat – 38 g.

Carbs – 15 g.

Chicken Drumsticks with Potatoes & Veggies

Preparation Time: 10 minutes

Cooking Time: 40 minutes

Servings: 4

Ingredients:

4 potatoes, peeled and quartered

4 cups water

2 lemons, zested and juiced

1 tbsp olive oil

2 tsp fresh oregano

1 tsp red pepper flakes

Salt and black pepper to taste

2 serrano peppers, stemmed, cored, chopped

4 boneless skinless chicken drumsticks

3 tbsp finely chopped parsley

1 cup packed watercress

1 cucumber, sliced

½ cup cherry tomatoes, quartered

¼ cup kalamata olives, pitted

¼ cup hummus

¼ cup feta cheese, crumbled

Lemon wedges, for serving

Directions:

In the cooker, add water and potatoes. Set trivet over them. In a baking bowl, mix lemon juice, olive oil, black pepper, oregano, zest, salt, and red pepper flakes. Add chicken drumsticks in the marinade and stir to coat.

Set the bowl with chicken on the trivet in the inner pot. Seal the lid, select Poultry and cook on High for 15 minutes. Do a quick release.

Take out the bowl with chicken and the trivet from the pot. Drain potatoes and add parsley and salt.

Divide the potatoes between four serving plates and top with watercress, cucumber slices, hummus, cherry tomatoes, chicken, olives, and feta cheese.

Garnish with lemon wedges to serve.

Nutrition:

Calories – 735

Protein – 67 g.

Fat – 45 g.

Carbs – 23 g.

Lebanese-Style Chicken with Fresh Couscous

Preparation Time: 10 minutes

Cooking Time: 40 minutes

Servings: 4

Ingredients:

4 chicken thighs

2 tbsp za'atar mix

1 tbsp ground sumac

Salt and black pepper to taste

2 tbsp butter

2 ½ cups chicken stock, divided

1 onion, chopped

1 garlic clove, minced

1 ½ cups couscous

Juice from 1 lemon

Fresh parsley, chopped

Directions:

Season the chicken with salt, sumac, za'atar, and pepper.

Melt butter on Sauté and sear the chicken in batches for 5 minutes per batch until lightly browned. Set aside. Into the cooker, add ¼ cup chicken stock to deglaze the pan, scrape the bottom to get rid of any browned bits of food. Add garlic and onion to the stock; cook for 3 minutes until soft.

Add the remaining chicken stock into the pan; add lemon juice and couscous. Add in chicken. Make sure to lock the lid and cook on High Pressure for 5 minutes. Naturally release the pressure for 5 minutes. Take the couscous and chicken to a serving plate; and garnish with parsley.

Nutrition:

Calories – 720

Protein – 63 g.

Fat – 42 g.

Carbs – 27 g.

Tasty Chicken Breasts with Barbeque Sauce

Preparation Time: 5 minutes

Cooking Time: 20 minutes

Servings: 6

Ingredients:

2 pounds boneless skinless chicken breasts

1 tsp salt

1 ½ cups barbecue sauce

1 small onion, minced

1 cup carrots, chopped

4 garlic cloves

Directions:

Rub salt onto chicken and place inside the instant pot. Add onion, carrots, garlic and barbeque sauce. Toss the chicken to coat. Seal the lid, press Poultry and cook on High for 15 minutes. Do a quick release. To shred chicken, use two forks and stir into the sauce.

Nutrition:

Calories – 655

Protein – 49 g.

Fat – 33.5 g.

Carbs – 14.7 g.

Friday Chicken & Avocado Fajitas

Preparation Time: 10 minutes

Cooking Time: 30 minutes

Servings: 4

Ingredients:

4 chicken breasts, boneless and skinless

1 taco seasoning

1 tbsp olive oil

1 (24-ounce) can diced tomatoes

3 bell peppers, julienned

1 shallot, chopped

4 garlic cloves, minced

juice of 1 lemon

Salt and pepper to taste

4 flour tortillas

2 tbsp cilantro, chopped

1 avocado, sliced

Directions:

In a bowl, mix taco seasoning and chicken until evenly coated. Warm oil on Sauté mode.

Sear chicken for 2 minutes per side until browned. To the chicken, add tomatoes, cilantro, shallot, lemon juice, garlic, and bell peppers; Season with pepper and salt.

Seal the lid, press Poultry and cook for 4 minutes on High Pressure. Release the Pressure quickly. Move the bell peppers and chicken to tortillas. Add avocado slices and serve.

Nutrition:

Calories – 660

Protein – 51 g.

Fat – 33 g.

Carbs – 14 g.

Thai Red Duck

Preparation Time: 10 minutes

Cooking Time: 40 minutes

Servings: 4

Ingredients:

1 tablespoon Thai red curry paste

Zest and juice of 1 fresh lime

2 pounds duck breast

1 tablespoon olive oil

1/2 teaspoon black peppercorns, crushed

1 teaspoon cayenne pepper

1 teaspoon sea salt

4 garlic cloves, minced

2 thyme sprigs, chopped

2 rosemary sprigs, chopped

1 cup light coconut milk

1/2 cup chicken broth, preferably homemade

1/4 small pack coriander, roughly chopped

Directions:

Combine the red curry paste with the lime zest and juice; rub the mixture all over the duck breast and leave it to marinate for 30 minutes.

Press the "Sauté" button and heat the oil until sizzling. Cook the duck breast until slightly brown on both sides. Then, season the duck breasts with the peppercorns, cayenne pepper, and salt. Add the garlic, thyme, rosemary, coconut milk, and chicken broth.

Secure the lid. Choose the "Poultry" mode and cook for 15 minutes at High pressure. Once done cooking, use a quick pressure release; carefully remove the lid.

Garnish with chopped coriander and serve warm. Bon appétit!

Nutrition:

Calories – 467

Protein – 47.6 g.

Fat – 27.8 g.

Carbs – 6.8 g.

Conclusion

When you are on a diet trying to lose weight or manage a condition, you will be strictly confined to follow an eating plan. Such plans often place numerous demands on individuals: food may need to be boiled, other foods are forbidden, permitting you only to eat small portions and so on.

On the other hand, a lifestyle such as the Mediterranean diet is entirely stress-free. It is easy to follow because there are almost no restrictions. There is no time limit on the Mediterranean diet because it is more of a lifestyle than a diet. You do not need to stop at some point but carry on for the rest of your life. The foods that you eat under the Mediterranean model include unrefined cereals, white meats, and the occasional dairy products.

The Mediterranean lifestyle, unlike other diets, also requires you to engage with family and friends and share meals together. It has been noted that communities around the Mediterranean spend between one and two hours enjoying their meals. This kind of bonding between family members or friends helps bring people closer together, which helps foster closer bonds hence fewer cases of depression, loneliness, or stress, all of which are precursors to chronic diseases.

You will achieve many benefits using the Instant Pot Pressure Cooker. These are just a few instances you will discover in your Mediterranean-style recipes:

Pressure cooking means that you can (on average) cook meals 75% faster than boiling/braising on the stovetop or baking and roasting in a conventional oven.

This is especially helpful for vegan meals that entail the use of dried beans, legumes, and pulses. Instead of pre-soaking these ingredients for hours before use, you can pour them directly into the Instant Pot, add water, and pressure cook these for several minutes. However, always follow your recipe carefully since they have been tested for accuracy.

Nutrients are preserved. You can use your pressure-cooking techniques using the Instant Pot to ensure the heat is evenly and quickly distributed. It is not essential to immerse the food into the water. You will provide plenty of water in the cooker for efficient steaming. You will also be saving the essential vitamins and minerals. The food won't become oxidized by the exposure of air or heat. Enjoy those fresh green veggies with their natural and vibrant colors.

The cooking elements help keep the foods fully sealed, so the steam and aromas don't linger throughout your entire home. That is a plus, especially for items such as cabbage, which throws out a distinctive smell.

You will find that beans and whole grains will have a softer texture and will have an improved taste. The meal will be cooked consistently since the Instant Pot provides even heat distribution.

You'll also save tons of time and money. You will be using much less water, and the pot is fully insulated, making it more energy-efficient when compared to boiling or steaming your foods on the stovetop. It is also less expensive than using a microwave, not to mention how much more flavorful the food will be when prepared in the Instant Pot cooker.

You can delay the cooking of your food items so you can plan ahead of time. You won't need to stand around as you await your meal. You can reduce the cooking time by reducing the 'hands-on' time. Just leave for work or a day of activities, and you will come home to a special treat. In a nutshell, the Instant Pot is:

Easy To Use

Healthy recipes for the entire family are provided.

You can make authentic one-pot recipes in your Instant Pot.

If you forget to switch on your slow cooker, you can make any meal done in a few minutes in your Instant Pot.

You can securely and smoothly cook meat from frozen.

It's a laid-back way to cook. You don't have to watch a pan on the stove or a pot in the oven.

The pressure cooking procedure develops delicious flavors swiftly.

CPSIA information can be obtained
at www.ICGtesting.com
Printed in the USA
BVHW011137080421
604414BV00020B/81